NO NONSENSE PARENTING GUIDE

PREGNANCY, BIRTH AND BONDING

OTHER NO NONSENSE PARENTING GUIDES

Fathering
Your Growing Baby
Feeding Your Baby
Play and Learn
The Working Mother
Raising A Happy Baby
Your Baby's Health and Safety

OTHER NO NONSENSE GUIDES

Real Estate Guides
Financial Guides
Legal Guides
Career Guides
Success Guides
Health Guides
Cooking Guides
Wine Guides

Pregnancy, Birth and Bonding

A GUIDE FOR THE MOTHER-TO-BE

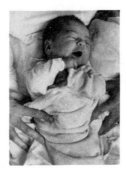

Carolyn T. Chubet

LONGMEADOW PRESS

PREGNANCY, BIRTH AND BONDING

Copyright © 1988 by Carolyn T. Chubet

No Nonsense Parenting Guide is a trademark controlled by
Longmeadow Press.

ISBN 0-681-40450-7

Printed in the United States of America

0 9 8 7 6 5 4 3 2 1

PREPARED FOR LONGMEADOW PRESS BY
IRENA CHALMERS BOOKS, INC.
MANAGING EDITOR: Jean Atcheson
COVER DESIGN: Karen Skelton
ART DIRECTION & DESIGN: Helene Berinsky
PICTURE RESEARCHER: Lisa Sorensen
TYPESETTING: ComCom, Allentown, Pennsylvania
PRODUCTION SERVICES: William S. Konecky Associates, New York

Cover photograph © 1988 Penny Gentieu

Contents

For John and Charlie

ACKNOWLEDGMENTS

With thanks to Judy Kay Morris, R.N., Certified Nurse-Midwife with the Sharon, Connecticut, Ob/Gyn Associates, who read my manuscript and offered many valuable comments.

Introduction

There is no "right" time to have a baby.

Women today make a variety of decisions about having children. Some choose to wait until their thirties, firmly establishing their careers before starting a family. These women have their babies and either continue their careers, or leave work and decide to stay at home. Others choose to begin having babies early in their twenties and then add on a career after their children have grown up. Still others have their babies early and manage a career at the same time; other women make raising a family their career.

Making a decision such as this requires you to look at your goals, priorities, realities and prospects. You will make the best choice when you have analyzed all the pros and cons, ifs and buts in *your* life. Be confident in your choice and try not to compare it to the decisions others make. Everybody is different, with individual considerations to think about. No one person has *the* answer.

Once the philosophical decision has been made to start up the baby factory, the final decision is left to nature. Conception usually occurs within a year's time, and sometimes it happens right away. If you conceive soon after you decide, or if the baby comes along by chance, you may very well wish there had been more time. But little by little you will adjust your life to accommodate the idea of a new baby. It is hard to think of anything on a list of must-do's that cannot be amended, postponed or fitted into your new life as a parent.

The humble but crucial drama of becoming a parent begins the moment you suspect you are pregnant. You have just missed your period, and perhaps feel nauseous and tired, two common complaints in the early going. Your suspicions send you to the corner drugstore to buy a home pregnancy test kit or to your gynecologist for testing. These days, current clinic urine tests can give positive results only three days after a missed period. Your test results are affirmative and a thrill runs through you. You rush to tell your mate as soon as possible.

The realization that a baby is on the way turns the right-side-up world completely upside down for you both. Only a moment ago it was just the two of you; now you are a conglomerate, at least in your mind's eye. Even if the baby is planned, even if you have thought long and hard about having a family, it is not unusual to have some misgivings.

Suddenly the future is now, ready or not. You feel quite differently, as Cinderella must have when her fairy godmother gave her the nod. You are amazed that when you look in the mirror you see the same person as before. The change is major, but it is not yet apparent to others, either. When you go into public now, no one notices that you are different.

Thinking about the future baby is both exciting and alarming. After all, this is not a sweater to knit or a loaf of bread for the oven. When this project is complete, it will be a new human being. A pregnant woman has an important assignment with a long-term agreement attached to it. Uncertainties about your ability to raise the baby well may multiply. "How will I" and "What if" situations are uninvited, unwelcome guests that pop into your brain.

Relax. Take comfort that you are eager to do the job well, a necessary prerequisite for any successful venture, including parenting. Your earnest enthusiasm will carry you and the baby through any rough terrain that lies ahead. Stop a minute and think about all the babies you know who have made it to adulthood safe and sound!

You have ample time to get ready and, in fact, after nine months you will be anxious to have that baby in your arms. An advantage of pregnancy is that it buys you some time to prepare for the baby's arrival intellectually and emotionally as well as physically. Part of this preparation will be reading this book and others written about babies; other essentials will be consulting a doctor and planning your baby's birth, first home and wardrobe.

This book is in no way an exhaustive, detailed account of exactly what happens. You will find that in many other sources. What we have tried to offer here is a sort of blueprint of your transition into motherhood. We shall look at nutrition and exercise, how you are likely to feel, and your relationship with your mate. We will go through the decisions to address before the baby comes and discuss the momentous events of labor and childbirth. And, finally, in Chapter 5 we will bring the baby home at last.

CHAPTER 1

The First Three Months: Basic Training

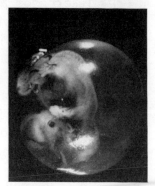

An eight-week embryo in the amniotic sac

Your Baby Is Being Formed Now

Development in the first three months is critical. The fertilized egg grows at an astonishing rate, laying out the basic plan that will be carried out over the next nine months. By six weeks, just four weeks after the first period has been missed, the embryo has already managed to form the beginnings of hands and feet with buds that will be fingers and toes, and sketched outlines of the heart and skeleton. At six weeks, although the baby is tiny, only about a half inch long, it already has begun to assemble the body that will someday throw a tantrum or hug your leg.

Thirty-four weeks later, only 40 weeks after conception,

your baby will be ready for birth. One of the first things you'll want to find out is when that is going to be. To calculate your estimated due date (EDD), or due date, count back three months from the first day of your last period and add seven days. And remember, your EDD is only an estimate of when your baby will be born. There's a two-week window before and after that day. Your baby could choose any of those days, too.

By the end of the third month, the baby is four times the size it was at six weeks—about two inches long. By 12 weeks the fetus is completely formed. The tiny factory in the womb has been busy growing bones and shaping fingers, toes, eyes and ears. Miraculously, the baby's face appears. Meanwhile, the baby's liver and spleen are on the job making blood cells, the heart is beating and tiny muscles have begun to do their exercises, too.

The baby's sex, of course, was determined at the moment the sperm fused with the egg. Now the interior reproductive organs begin to take shape and boy and girl babies have recognizable external organs too, molded from what were formerly folds of near-identical tissue. For the purposes of this chapter, we'll assume the baby to be a boy. In subsequent chapters, we will alternate the baby's sex. After all, boys and girls are born in just about equal numbers— fortunately!

You Have Work to Do, Too

The only source of energy for all this activity is you, the pregnant mother. The baby needs a steady stream of many nutrients to fuel the formation and growth of his tiny body. So from the very beginning he needs you to eat a balanced,

THE 1974 RECOMMENDED DIETARY ALLOWANCES (RDA)

RDA	Nonpregnant		Pregnant	
Energy	2,000	calories	2,300	calories
Protein	44	g	74	g
Vitamin A	800	mg	1,000	mg
Vitamin D	5	mcg	10	mcg
Vitamin E	8	mg	10	mg
Vitamin C	60	mg	80	mg
Folic Acid	400	mg	800	mg
Niacin	13	mg	15	mg
Riboflavin	1.2	mg	1.5	mg
Thiamine	1	mg	1.4	mg
Vitamin B6	2	mg	2.6	mg
Vitamin B12	3	mcg	4	mcg
Calcium	800	mg	1,200	mg
Phosphorus	800	mg	1,200	mg
Iodine	150	mcg	175	mcg
Iron	18	mg	48	mg
Magnesium	300	mg	450	mg
Zinc	15	mg	20	mg

SOURCE: Issued by the Food and Nutrition Board of the National Academy of Science.

nutritional diet. (If you are not pregnant yet, but hope to be soon, you can give your baby the best possible start if you begin eating well now.)

A pregnant woman needs more of every nutrient than her nonpregnant counterpart. She must add 30 more grams of protein, double the amount of folic acid and

```
┌─────────────────────────────────────────────────┐
│                   DAILY MENU                    │
│                                                 │
│  Milk or yogurt (or the equivalent in   4 cups or 1 quart │
│     cottage cheese or other cheeses)            │
│  Meat, poultry, fish, beans             3 servings │
│  Dark green and yellow vegetables       1/2 cup │
│  Citrus fruits or juice                 1/2 cup │
│  Other fruits and vegetables            1 cup   │
│  Grains (bread and cereals)             5 servings │
│  Water and fluids                       6–8 glasses │
└─────────────────────────────────────────────────┘
```

almost triple the iron to her diet. Often medical advisers suggest prenatal vitamins to supplement the diet. You should check with your health team before adding any vitamin to your daily routine.

The food you eat should be spread out among four basic food groups: milk products, meats and fish, vegetables and fruits, grains. Luckily there is a wide variety of foods in each category to choose from, enough to satisfy even the most delicate pregnant stomach. As soon as possible, you should ask your obstetrician to give you a dietary plan tailored to your individual needs.

GIVE BABY THE BEST CHANCE FOR A GOOD START

- No cigarettes
- No alcohol
- No recreational drugs
- No prescription or nonprescription drugs, without consulting your physician or health adviser
- Caffeine in moderation (but you may want to abstain as it may interfere with sleeping)

Gaining Weight: Eating for Two Doesn't Mean Eating Twice as Much

No one really knows exactly how much weight should be gained during pregnancy. Some findings show that, other things being equal, women of normal weight before pregnancy who gain between 24 and 30 pounds, overweight women who gain 15 to 24 pounds, and underweight women who gain as many as 30 pounds, are more likely to have a successful pregnancy.

Unless you are vastly underweight, you must remember that after the baby is born you will want to take off the weight that you put on in your pregnancy. Too often excess weight gain stubbornly hangs on—and on.

Despite their doctors' recommendations, some women gain more than 30 pounds, and though some successfully lose the excess weight after childbirth, many others retain the extra baggage. When the next pregnancy begins, they start out heavier than they should be, and then they repeat

HOW MUCH A SAMPLE PREGNANCY WEIGHS

Baby	7.5 lbs.
Placenta	2 lbs.
Amniotic fluid	2 lbs.
Maternal blood volume	4 lbs.
Uterus, breast tissue	4 lbs.
Extracellular fluid	4 lbs.
Maternal fat stores	2 lbs.
Total	25.5 lbs.

the process, adding on more and more weight. Nor is pregnancy the time to try to lose any pounds, if you are overweight.

Whatever your physique, most authorities say you should gain weight steadily, but gradually. As a general guide, you might think about gaining half a pound a week during the first 20 weeks and about one pound a week during the last 20 weeks, for a total of 30 pounds. The number of calories you can consume to achieve this slow, even increase depends on you, your metabolism and your level of activity and exercise.

Generally speaking, if you sit at a desk during the day and are a regular couch potato by night, you only need about 300 extra calories a day during pregnancy. If you exercise regularly, you will need more fuel for the fire. How much you need depends on the type of exercise and how long you exercise for. As a broad suggestion, you may add 200 more calories to your diet on days when you exercise for half an hour. If your weight gain then falls below normal, add more calories; if it rises too high, you should cut back accordingly.

Exercising: Exercise Caution, Too

Playing active sports and exercising while pregnant is a tricky business and the medical community remains uncertain about what is safe during pregnancy. Many doctors worry about moderate or heavy exercise interfering with the oxygen flow to the baby, which would retard his growth in the uterus. This and other real concerns about the baby's well-being lead many doctors to feel that only sports such as swimming and walking are safe in pregnancy.

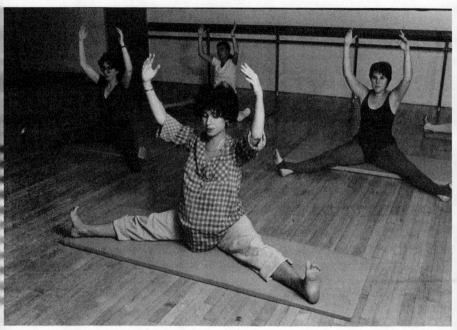

Prenatal exercise class helps some women keep in shape throughout pregnancy.

In addition, your body is changing subtly. During pregnancy hormones relax the cartilage in the pelvis, in preparation for childbirth. But this also makes the pelvis less stable, so you are more susceptible to injury and falls. You also may find yourself feeling dizzy more easily than you did. (Chapter 3 tells more about how you may feel during your pregnancy.)

So before you work up a sweat of any kind, consult your health-care team for guidance. You must consult with a professional now, even if you have been following a certain regimen for years. Your body is not the same as it was before you were pregnant and you have a fragile guest in your womb whose needs *must* come first.

Morning Sickness: Now for the Good News

If you are often nauseated at the smell, sight or thought of certain foods, you already know the bad news. You have lots of company: About half of all pregnant women have nausea and vomiting in the first three months. No one really knows what causes morning sickness, but a likely culprit is the increased hormonal activity in your body.

The hormones your body makes now are busy helping the baby take form during these crucial first months. Some findings show that a very high hormonal level or the resultant hormonal imbalance may cause the nausea of morning sickness; this may be seen as a good sign for the pregnancy. But it should be stressed that the absence of morning sickness is by no means a bad sign for the pregnancy. It is certainly a lot pleasanter for the mother-to-be.

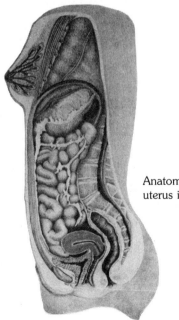

Anatomical view, showing the uterus in a nonpregnant state

- Put crackers by your bed to eat before you raise your head from the pillow
- Get out of bed slowly
- Eat small, easily prepared meals frequently
- Avoid fried, greasy or highly seasoned foods
- Choose bland food like chicken, baked potatoes and rice
- Take small sips of liquids such as apple juice or carbonated beverages
- Get plenty of fresh air and avoid hot, stuffy rooms

While you have been feeling terrible, the placenta that will soon take over as the baby's *in utero* life-support system has been under construction. Finally, after three months of preparation, it is ready to take over the hormone production business. As the placenta assumes its duties, you feel a hundred times better. Luckily, each subsequent pregnancy is different and sickness may not bother you the next time.

Miscarriage

Miscarriage is nature's way of saying that there was a problem with a particular pregnancy. Despite the logic of this natural ending to a pregnancy that cannot succeed, coping with losing a fetus in the early months of pregnancy is difficult. When a woman miscarries, she rides an emotional roller coaster. She begins the pregnancy in excited euphoria and ends it in mental anguish and depression, or when the outcome is final, she may even feel relieved of the worry that started when the bleeding first began.

About one in five documented pregnancies end in spontaneous abortion, the medical term for miscarriage. Doctors suspect that many more occur, but they happen so close to the menstrual period that they are not detected.

An early sign of possible miscarriage is bleeding, usually accompanied by cramps. About one-third of women will have some degree of spotting during pregnancy. Miscarriages usually start and end quickly (within 24 to 48 hours) whereas benign spotting may go on for weeks. If you experience some bleeding in the first few months, do not be overly alarmed, but be sure to notify your doctor right away. Half of the pregnancies that are threatened with bleeding go to full term. It is also important to note that babies born after bleeding has threatened the pregnancy are just as likely to be normal as any others.

Though there is no proof that exercise heightens the risk of miscarriage or stops it from occurring, usually the doctor's advice is to rest as much as possible and to cut back on such activities as sex. If the bleeding stops, the outlook is very promising.

SOME POSSIBLE CAUSES OF EARLY MISCARRIAGE

Smoking	Abnormalities of the uterus
Genetic defect, virus or infection	A poor womb environment caused by faulty "nesting" of the embryo or insufficient production of progesterone, the growth hormone
Malnutrition	
Exposure to toxic agents	
Physical trauma	

Telling the World: You May Want to Wait

As the previous section on miscarriage suggests, there are good reasons to keep your pregnancy a secret for a while.

Until the possibility of losing the baby is unlikely (90 percent of all miscarriages occur in the first three months), it may be best to keep quiet. If the worst should happen, you would have to tell all those people you have lost a baby, a task that you would surely not relish. In addition, telling others about a baby on the way increases your own excitement level, which will make your disappointment all the more severe if by some chance the pregnancy should end prematurely.

On the other hand, some women want the world to know immediately. These women reason that the great majority of pregnancies do *not* end in miscarriage and they are therefore unwilling to hold themselves back from sharing the joy.

If miscarriage does occur, there are support groups in many communities to help you through the adjustment period.

You've Made It!

The beginning of pregnancy is a crucial time for the baby: Chemistry and biology are bubbling along, building the framework of a human life. Inside your uterus your baby is following the time-honored formula for extending human history. For your part, as this baby's mother, you have signed an invisible contract to nurture and protect a new life from its inception. Let's turn now to the physical and emotional slumps and surges that accompany even the most normal pregnancies.

CHAPTER 2

Life
Changes

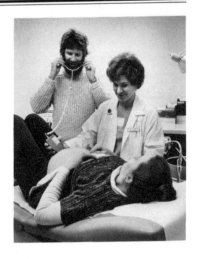

Now that you have made it through the first trimester of pregnancy and the threat of miscarriage has faded, we can expand our horizon to include all nine months of pregnancy and discuss the physical and mental changes to watch out for. As morning sickness ends and your energy level perks up a bit, other things begin to happen as you get further into pregnancy. In this chapter we will look at some ways to help you cope with them.

If by some chance you missed the sections in Chapter 1 on eating and exercise guidelines to follow throughout these very special nine months, please go back and read them now.

The Inside Story

Before we talk about you and your concerns in pregnancy, let's peek inside and see what the baby is doing during these next six months. In the second trimester the baby develops her brain, a physical process that continues until she is 18 months old. At the same time she forms her bone structure, and begins to change cartilage into bone. By the sixth month the baby has grown to be about a foot long and weighs more than a pound. She likes to do her exercises and kicks you regularly, turning a cartwheel now and then to break the monotony. When she is tuckered out, she may suck her thumb.

In her last three months in the womb, baby makes a final growth spurt, gaining a half pound to a full pound each

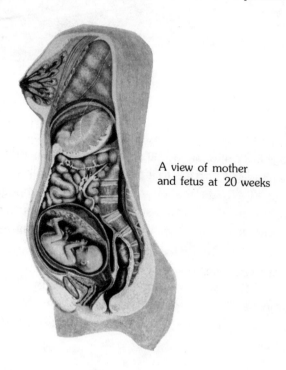

A view of mother
and fetus at 20 weeks

week and growing about eight inches. She gets the finishing touches, including important antibodies against disease and a protective covering for her skin. She has much less room for calisthenics now, and settles into the head-down position (if she is feet-first at birth, she will be in a "breech" position and a cesarean birth may be suggested).

If a baby is born in the middle of this trimester, she has about a 90 percent chance of survival. These days babies born early have a much better chance than they did two decades ago. Neonatal intensive care units have learned a lot about helping the tiniest babies learn to breathe and eat with systems that have not had the final weeks they need to develop. Full-term babies use these final weeks to finish getting ready and average about 20 inches long and weigh about 7.7 or 7.8 pounds (depending on the sex of the baby; boys are usually slightly heavier).

Maternity Clothes: Wait to the Last Minute

As the baby grows, so will your waistline. You should delay the switch into maternity clothes until the clothes you used to wear are truly uncomfortable. It is wise to wait because women usually find they are heartily sick of their maternity wardrobe by the end of their pregnancy and are dismayed to find they do not fit into their regular clothes after the baby is born. If you postpone the change, you will shorten the time of choosing from what will rapidly be an all-too-familiar wardrobe.

WHAT TO BUY (SEW OR BORROW IF YOU CAN)
Your lifestyle and the weather of the six-month season ahead will dictate the clothes you need. Current fashions

offer a wide range of loose-fitting, upbeat clothes that will fit pregnant women, in addition to the maternity wear that is available in specialty shops. Mixing and matching colors will help you get the most mileage from your selections. If you plan to work during your pregnancy, you may need to add more dresses or suits to the list offered above.

Your Wardrobe Isn't All That Changes

Pregnancy shows itself in many ways other than your thickening middle:

YOUR BREASTS

These become sensitive early in pregnancy. Later they are engorged with blood and swollen because the hormones estrogen and progesterone are busily preparing them for nursing. By the middle of the second trimester they are ready to feed the baby with the special fluid called colostrum that is the forerunner of the milk supply for the nursing baby. A good support bra will help to ease the heaviness of extra-large breasts. (A nursing bra should be the same size as your bra in pregnancy and have an easy open/close cup fastener like Velcro.)

APPETITE

The appetite and tastes for certain foods often change during pregnancy. No one really knows why women commonly crave foods that may be very sour, salty, bitter or sweet. Most experts agree that these cravings are not linked to dietary need. The amount of indulgence you can allow yourself depends on what you crave. You can be more permissive if you are suddenly crazy about leafy green salads, which are relatively low in calories and healthy to eat. Beware of empty calories. Unless eaten only occasionally in very small amounts, highly salted, very acidic or high caloric foods are just plain trouble.

MOOD SWINGS

Feeling happy one minute and weepy the next is extremely common in pregnancy. Without much warning you can switch from feeling excited about your baby to being ambivalent about her, or even downright resentful. You may become an emotional Vesuvius spewing anxiety attacks, identity crises and short-tempered remarks. Your mate, who is probably having his own identity crises, catches the brunt of it. If you understand that these emotional zigzags are normal, caused mostly by hormonal imbalances in pregnancy, it will help you and your husband get through the bad times. Remember that your hormones are in the driver's seat these days and try to keep a sense of humor. Humor heals frayed nerve endings and often can stop an unnecessary argument dead in its tracks.

Another way to get away from moodiness is to decide that you need to reward yourself for a job well done. In addition, an understanding relationship with your husband will help get you both through the emotional minefield of being pregnant. We'll discuss ways of achieving both these goals later in the chapter.

SLEEP

This most important function can be fitful, disrupted by nightmares and by an increasingly squeezed bladder demanding relief. Bad dreams about losing the baby or having a difficult childbirth are common, particularly in the last weeks of pregnancy. Nightmares like these are understandable: People often dream about what they fear most.

Frequent trips to the bathroom cannot really be remedied, because of the need to drink fluids in pregnancy. If you think about it, however, getting up in the middle of the night for the bathroom is actually good training for night duty later on when your newborn baby wakes to be fed.

INSOMNIA

This usually comes in the last few weeks when the baby is getting heavy and exerts pressure that may make it difficult for you to find a comfortable sleeping position. If she waits to do her gymnastics at 2:00 A.M. you may find it hard to sleep through gym class. If you add to all this a few worries to stew about in the middle of the night, you have a perfect recipe for insomnia.

Some remedies: Drink a small glass of warm milk and try a warm bath before bed. When you go to bed, lie on your left side, knees apart, with a pillow under your right knee to improve the circulation. Try different pillows or add others. Read a boring book. If you wake, try a little more milk and read some more of that book. If all else fails, nap when you can.

Bodily Displeasures

Some women sail through pregnancy with a minimum of physical discomforts. The rest of us mortals are likely to suffer a variety of complaints with varying intensities. Some problems can be helped, others must be tolerated. At no time should you take medicines without first checking with your medical adviser; always check at once if any symptoms start to worry you.

Pamper Yourself

There is a myth floating about that pregnancy is a wonderful time. For most women it isn't. Too often women believe the fiction of maternal bliss which catapults them into an almost deified role. To get this ideal role to fit, women must

DISCOMFORTS: SOME POSSIBLE CAUSES AND REMEDIES

Complaint	Possible Causes	Possible Remedies
Backache	Uterus exerting pressure on lower back; ligaments or joints loosening	Better posture, massage, heating pad, warm shower; proper sleep position on side, knees up
Constipation	Intestines blocked by uterus; bowel-needed water absorbed elsewhere; hormonal activity blocking digestion	Drink extra water; eat bran and fiber, prunes; take a walk
Tiredness	Sedative power of progesterone; feature of early pregnancy before placenta takes over; natural feature of late pregnancy	Listen to your body, sleep and rest as much as possible; take another walk!
Heartburn/ indigestion	Digestion slowed by hormonal activity; pressure from enlarged uterus	Avoid trouble foods; eat small meals; sip carbonated fluids
Hemorrhoids	Constipation and straining; hormonal activity strains bowel movements, dilates rectal veins	Avoid constipation; get off your feet, with hips raised; try an ice pack or use refrigerated Tucks

Complaint	Possible Causes	Possible Remedies
Muscle cramp/ charley horse	Fatigue; calcium imbalance; sluggish circulation; not enough salt; pointing toes	Warm bath, light massage; give the hurt muscle rapid massage; pull foot toward you
Shooting pains	Pelvic ligaments, bones and nerves getting ready for baby	Try the Kegel exercise (the perineal squeeze)
Swelling/edema	Fluid retention (the body becomes a giant sponge)	Watch salt in the diet; drink water (not soda); lie down on left side, with legs raised on a cushion
Varicose veins	Hormone activity in muscles; excessive weight gain; heredity	Lie down on left side, with feet up; don't cross legs; wear support stockings; watch your weight
Dizzy spells	Brain suffers decrease in oxygen-rich blood, now diverted to uterus	Sit down quickly, put head to knees and take deep breaths; eat regularly

gloss over the difficult aspects of pregnancy—no small job, if you look at the laundry list of changes and discomforts described above.

A woman who falls for this myth knows she is supposed to be euphoric and blissful. But she is not; indeed, she is prey to violent emotional changes. Her mood, if anything, is blacker because her pregnancy is not a storybook experience; she feels she's been had.

Now suppose we change her perspective, and suggest that she looks at her pregnancy as hard work for which she should be rewarded. Suddenly that black mood lightens up and everything looks more hopeful. It is important, however, that we also get her to explain to everyone close to her—and especially her husband—the new rules of the game. For if the people around do not understand, the clouds may darken ominously.

Rewards can be anything, as long as they are valued and don't add extra weight or put undue strain on the pocketbook. You can find large and small ways to pat yourself on the back (this is not meant to be a choice between a small or a large banana split!). Take a moment to ponder what would appeal to you. Perhaps a beauty make-over or a

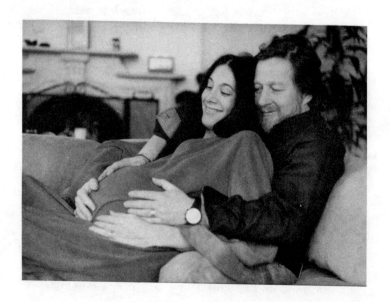

professional manicure, a long-distance call to a faraway friend or a special pair of earrings would give you a boost. The reward does not have to be a trip to a Caribbean island—though that might be nice, too.

There is another very good reason for treating yourself well: You will not have much time to do it later on. Your baby, when she comes, is going to take up all of your time and sap most of your energy. But there is time now before the baby comes to do something that you have always wanted to do, but have postponed for some reason. If you have an idea in mind, consult with your doctor and your checkbook, and if you get a green light, go for it!

Communicate with Your Mate

Your husband is going through changes, too. In pregnancy you begin to undertake the transformation from being a couple into being a family, a difficult, even painful transition. Before your baby is even born, she intrudes herself into the intimate world of your togetherness as a couple. She jeopardizes the balance of emotional give-and-take you established when you joined together. The baby's insistent thumps at your rib cage force you to redefine who you are. Both partners feel disoriented and struggle to adjust to the new situation.

Take heart. Honest communication and mutual trust will help guide you through the emotional tangle of becoming parents. Each of you must understand what is happening to the other. In the *Pamper Yourself* section, we have just said that you need to explain your predicament in the pregnancy to your husband. And as night follows day, the man in your life must also be willing and able to express his hopes, doubts and anxieties to *you.* Once you are communicating fully, mutual trust will follow and you can begin to relax and enjoy the remaining months alone together while Baby is with you, but still under wraps.

Sex in Pregnancy

Speaking of enjoying your mate, let us turn to the subject of sex life during pregnancy. Having a good sex life is vital, its power undeniable. Sexual intimacy and affection can be powerful allies to help you through the rough spots of your life together during these months of waiting for the baby. By definition sex is a special, pleasurable way to communicate feelings and needs, and at the same time a reward you both owe yourselves.

The trick is, of course, not to be too tired to enjoy it. Do not postpone sex until the last thing at night when one or both of you is too exhausted to care. Try first thing in the morning, before dinner or after a nap. Experiment, and make it a priority.

The medical community generally believes that in a normal pregnancy—one with no complications or special medical concerns—sexual intercourse can be unrestricted in the first two trimesters. Recommendations for the third trimester differ because doctors do not agree whether intercourse causes premature labor and they often worry about infection. Research by Masters and Johnson, the noted authorities on sex, shows that though coitus will probably not start labor, it may initiate or stimulate contractions if conditions are right for childbirth.

If for some reason your doctor bans intercourse, masturbation or other stimulation is usually also precluded, on the theory that any orgasm will stimulate the uterus to contract.

SEXUAL INTEREST DURING PREGNANCY

Stage of Pregnancy	Positive	Negative
First Trimester	Because no longer anxious to conceive, or because free from contraceptive use, more relaxed	Tired, nauseous and perhaps worried about miscarriage
Second Trimester	Increased blood flow to breasts and pelvis, increased lubrication (vaginal discharge) and elevated production of estrogen and steroids make some women feel erotically supercharged	More afraid of hurting baby because of awareness of his/her presence due to size and movements
Third Trimester	Sexual intimacy provides reassurance in relationship, particularly during final weeks, when expectant mother tends to feel more vulnerable and dependent	Fatigue, physical discomfort, awkwardness, feeling unattractive

SOURCE: *The Maternity Sourcebook,* by Matthew and Wendy Lesko (Warner Books, 1984).

But more and more experts agree that, in the absence of certain complications, you have the green light as long as it feels comfortable, until the last few weeks. As always, ask your medical team what they advise for you, and be sure to alert them to any bleeding or abdominal pain after sex.

In practice the pregnant couple will discover that the man above, woman below position must be abandoned in the second trimester. Two common alternatives put the woman above the man, or have the man entering the vagina from behind. In any case, ingenuity and a sense of humor will get you both through the awkwardness of trial and error.

In this chapter we have looked at the physical, emotional and psychological changes in pregnancy. We have decided that pregnancy is hard work that needs tender loving care as a reward. The care and nurturing of you and your husband must not be forgotten or neglected, as the baby worms her way into your hearts. In the next chapter we begin our plans for Labor Day (hint: it's not a holiday).

Decisions, Decisions

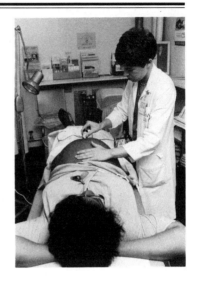

T here are amazing numbers of important choices to make during pregnancy, but don't let them overwhelm you because you feel you are a novice on the subject. As with any decision you make in life, find out the facts as best you can, ask experts for advice and weigh the pros and cons before you choose. If you take the big questions and break them down into little ones, the process will become much more manageable. Ponder each of the variables and decide which are most important to you. But be careful not to get bogged down in details. When you get to the end of the line, you will find you have accomplished a great deal.

THE BIRTH PLAN

This is the most important array of decisions for you now. Your plan for the baby's birth develops in stages as you approach the time for your delivery and grow in your understanding of what is best for you and the baby.

The Early Phase

In the beginning you should think about the medical team you want to guide you now and be on hand at childbirth. In addition, you should have an idea where you want to have your baby—in a hospital, at an alternative birth center or at home—before you sign on with a medical team, who will be affiliated with a particular institution. If you have chosen a hospital setting, you must consider which hospital in your area is best. But which comes first, the place of birth or the medical team? In fact, they come hand in hand, but one may be more important to you than the other, depending on your particular situation.

THE MEDICAL TEAM

If you have a gynecologist whom you like and trust who also delivers babies, then you are less likely to start from scratch looking for an obstetric team. But obstetrics is a different field from gynecology: Make sure that the obstetricians' philosophy of pregnancy and childbirth follows lines of thinking you are comfortable with.

If you find that you do not agree with your doctor, you may be forced to find another team. Or you may discover that the hospital your doctor is affiliated with does not offer the kind of environment for childbirth you want. Another reason which will force you to look around: Your doctor may not be a practicing obstetrician. Because of the high malpractice insurance fees for obstetrics, fewer doctors are delivering babies these days.

To evaluate the medical support system you have now, or as a starting place for finding a new one, take a blank sheet of paper and a pen. Jot down your ideas about what is important to you in a doctor and what you would like a hospital to offer. What you write will depend on your own situation; it will be a statement of your own medical and personal concerns. If you have a special problem, you may have to focus on finding a doctor who has expertise on the subject.

A SAMPLE DOCTOR AND HOSPITAL WISH LIST

DOCTOR

- **Up to date on the latest developments in pregnancy and childbirth**
- **Follows reasonable rules for cesarean birth**
- **Suggests minimal or no drugs during labor**
- **All members of the team share the primary doctor's childbirth philosophy**
- **Has friendly, respectful manner, is not condescending**
- **Believes in prepared childbirth**

HOSPITAL

- **Birthing rooms available**
- **Rooming-in**
- **Father can attend a cesarean birth**
- **Has the necessary emergency birth equipment and facilities**
- **Encourages breast-feeding and holding baby after delivery**

Your wish list may be very short or a detailed laundry list. Whichever it is, it will help you evaluate your current situa-

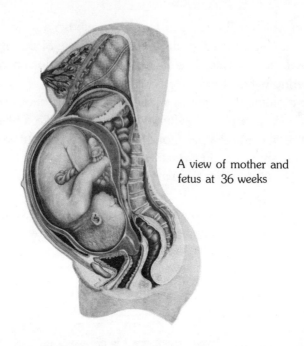

A view of mother and fetus at 36 weeks

tion and decide which teams to interview. You can also use these ideas to help you ask the right questions in an interview. The first draft of your ideal doctor and hospital criteria will probably undergo revision as you learn more about what is best for you and your baby. As you go about your research, listen to medical advisers you have confidence in, and to trusted friends with experience.

SOME HOSPITAL CONSIDERATIONS

You will not be able to satisfy every one of your wishes, so try to decide which are the most significant. If it is important to you to be able to move around during labor, this may be a key point to focus on. Hospital policies vary in permitting this, usually depending on the use of the fetal monitor (see page 62). Perhaps you want to have access to a birthing bed or chair which can pull apart and be adjusted to help you during labor and delivery. Or maybe you are most concerned about the hospital's rooming-in policy. When you finally decide who is going to help you and where, make sure you feel comfortable with your decision.

Alternatives: Certified Midwives and Birth Centers

CERTIFIED NURSE-MIDWIVES

These are professional registered nurses who have completed a rigorous educational program in caring for women and babies during pregnancy, childbirth and the postpartum period. To become certified they must pass national certification boards. Although these nurse-midwives independently manage the care of healthy women and newborns, each nurse-midwife is affiliated with a physician who is available for consultation or referral if needed.

They work in a variety of settings in private practice or are affiliated with a hospital, health maintenance organization (HMO) or birth center (see below). They handle routine prenatal care and monitor the pregnancy for any special concerns. If they suspect problems, they consult with the back-up physician; a high-risk pregnancy will always be turned over to the doctor.

Certified nurse-midwives are dedicated to the natural process of labor and birth and seek medical intervention only when necessary. They emphasize good nutrition and prepared childbirth training. Perhaps the most important advantage of having nurse-midwives on hand comes in labor and delivery: They will stay with you in labor and coach you through each contraction until the baby is born. Word-of-mouth referral is usually the best way to find a good certified nurse-midwife, but remember to check out the back-up physicians before you decide.

If you would like information on who is available in your area, write to the American College of Nurse-Midwives (1522 K St. NW, Suite 1120, Washington, DC 20005).

BIRTH CENTERS

Though the great majority of births still take place in hospitals, the number of alternative birth centers is steadily increasing. There is great debate about the advisability of using these centers, and safety is the central issue for both mother and baby. Few would argue that high-risk women should have their babies anywhere but in a hospital where they can be monitored and close to sophisticated emergency equipment should it be needed. Experts are divided, however, about the safety of birth centers for low-risk pregnancies.

These alternative centers vary considerably in their standards and practices, and at this writing there is no uniform mandatory licensing or accreditation procedure in place. If you are interested in getting information about birth centers and guidance on what to look for, write to the National Association of Childbearing Centers (Box 1, Route 1, Perkiomenville, PA 18074). This is a national organization that suggests guidelines and acts as an information clearinghouse for free-standing birth centers.

The Birth Plan: Phase Two

Now that we have considered the Who and the Where, we need to look at the How. The medical team and the place you choose to have your baby will help to determine the way your baby is born. But there is no way to know beforehand how your labor and childbirth will go. Every woman's labor is different and unpredictable.

Even though you cannot foretell what your childbirth experience will be, it *is* possible to plan or eliminate certain parts of the regular hospital labor and delivery routine. Shaving the pubic area, the enema, the automatic intravenous needle, the episiotomy (the incision that enlarges the vaginal opening to accommodate the baby's head at birth) and pain medication all may be discussed with your team. Other aspects of the routine are less negotiable. For example, most hospitals require a fetal monitor to record the baby's heartbeat as a check on how he is weathering the stress of each contraction, but there also may be a small window of flexibility at some hospitals which allows the mother to move about briefly without the monitor.

Childbirth Methods

A major decision that will shape your labor experience is the method of childbirth you choose to adopt. Your medical adviser may refer you to a childbirth instructor and suggest that you enroll in classes in your seventh or eighth month. Before signing up, it is important to find out whether you and the instructor have a rapport. Try to meet the instructor and talk about childbirth philosophy and what the classes will cover. If you are at all put off by the conversation, you will need to shop around for an instructor and classes that will teach what you want to learn.

There are several methods of childbirth available these days, usually with the name of the founder attached to them, but they all advocate preparation for childbirth and fall into one of two general categories. The psychopro-phylactic school, which usually is just referred to as Lamaze after the French physician who originated the method, seeks to deflect pain and teaches pain control through breathing, relaxation and distraction of the woman in labor. The Lamaze philosophy requires a labor coach to support and encourage the laboring woman. Lamaze teaches the couple to focus on one contraction at a time and assigns breathing patterns to each stage of labor.

The other is psychophysical. The major founders and their techniques in this category are Dr. Grantly Dick-Read's *Childbirth Without Fear,* Sheila Kitzinger's psycho-sexual theory and Dr. Robert Bradley's husband-coached childbirth. Though they differ in emphasis, these methods rely on creating a positive psychological state in the labor-ing woman to break the fear-tension-pain cycle. She is encouraged to tune into her body as it responds to the birthing process, aided by breathing and concentration techniques.

CHILDBIRTH CLASS TOPICS

- Information about birth, the stages of labor and nature of contractions in each stage
- Physical conditioning for labor and delivery
- Role of the labor coach
- Relaxation techniques
- Pain control techniques
- Positions in labor and delivery
- Comfort measures in labor, including pain medication
- Hospital policies and parents' options and rights
- Preparation for nursing

WHO WILL BE YOUR LABOR COACH?

Whatever method you decide to use, don't for a minute think you don't need a coach. You do. If your husband is reluctant or worried that he will not do a good enough job, try to get him to realize that it is *his* presence more than that of a strange labor nurse that will help you get through it. Find another man whom he knows and trusts who has been through the whole experience. Encourage him not to decide until he has attended some of the childbirth classes with you. You might alert the instructor to your problem so that your mate can get special attention.

If you are a single parent or your husband simply refuses to go along, you might seriously consider the certified nurse-midwife option we discussed earlier. Certified nurse-midwives are good at acting as your advocate and they have experiences to draw on to help you in labor. Another possibility is to ask a good friend, who has labored and delivered a baby and who is willing to be on 24-hour call, to go to childbirth classes with you and sit with you throughout labor.

Other Decisions to Make

In the course of your regular visits to the doctor during your pregnancy, you will be checked out carefully and the doctor will listen to your baby's heartbeat with a stethoscope. In the old days, though the mother would be offered the chance to "listen in" also, she had no tangible idea of the child in her womb. Now we have several ways of finding out very specific information about the fetus and checking whether everything is developing normally—long before the baby actually arrives.

VAGINAL BIRTH AFTER CESAREAN
(A NOTE FOR SECOND-TIME-AROUND MOTHERS)

Even if you had a cesarean birth in a previous pregnancy, you may still be able to labor and deliver your next baby vaginally. The American College of Obstetricians and Gynecologists has suggested guidelines for VBAC (pronounced *vee-bak*):

1. the reason for the previous cesarean must be nonrecurring (like fetal distress)
2. your cesarean incision is low transverse (horizontal)
3. your baby weighs less than eight and a half pounds, and is not in breech or feet-first position
4. this is not a multiple birth
5. there is continuous electronic fetal monitoring in labor
6. availability of an adequately staffed and equipped hospital if a cesarean birth must after all be performed

Even if you meet all your doctor's requirements for VBAC, you can still opt to have another cesarean birth and set up an appointment for the operation. There is an advantage in knowing when the baby is actually coming, because you are able to arrange your life and family schedule around a certain date. With a cesarean birth you also avoid the pain and exhaustion of labor, and epidural or local anesthesia will enable you to be awake at the birth of your baby.

While there is risk on either side (cesarean birth has the risk of surgery attached to it, while labor after cesarean carries with it a very slight chance of scar rupture), consider the advantages of vaginal birth. By laboring you

- are in control of the birth, rather than having a doctor performing an operation on you
- will be in touch with the baby
- will view the actual birth in the overhead mirror
- will be able to keep the baby free of anesthetic
- will have a speedy recovery, not usually associated with abdominal surgery.

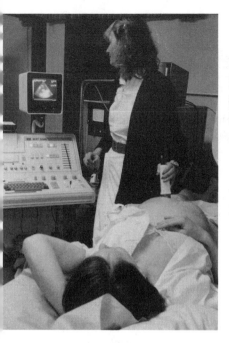

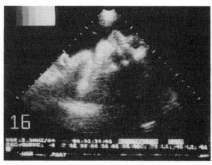

Scanning with ultrasound at 32 weeks. The screen (in closeup) shows the top of the baby's head.

SONOGRAMS

Ultrasound screening, which works much the same way as radar or sonar, bounces sound waves off the fetus which are translated into dots on a screen. High-tech equipment today enables doctors to examine the fetus for a variety of reasons, but the medical profession is not in total agreement about the routine use of sonograms for low-risk, trouble-free pregnancies. Nor do doctors agree about the advisability of repeated use on an individual. Controversy persists because little is known about the possible long-term effects on the baby.

If your medical team suggests a sonogram, be sure that there is a valid medical reason. If there is, the benefits of the test will likely outweigh the still unknown effects of a sonogram on your child.

AMNIOCENTESIS

This is the process of sampling a small amount of the amniotic fluid that surrounds the baby in the uterus by inserting a hollow needle through the abdomen into the amniotic sac. It is chiefly done if there is a possibility of chromosomal abnormalities such as Down's syndrome and other metabolic diseases. Doctors usually recommend an amniocentesis for women over 35, who have a higher likelihood of giving birth to a baby with Down's syndrome.

One valid reason for doing a sonogram, in fact, is as preparation for amniocentesis. An ultrasound "picture" taken just before the needle is inserted shows the position of the placenta and fetus so that accidental puncture can be avoided.

Amniocentesis is usually performed in the second trimester, somewhere between 15 and 19 weeks. The sample of amniotic fluid withdrawn contains fetal cells, and these cells are grown in a culture in a lab for two to six weeks before the results can be known.

Included in the results is the news of whether the baby is a boy or a girl. Parents may decide whether they want to be told the sex of their baby. Many parents are glad to know, because naming the baby and nursery preparations are simplified. Also it helps the parents visualize the future after the baby is born.

Legal and ethical arguments swirl about the amniocentesis. Doctors recommend the test under certain circumstances, but if the test shows abnormalities, it is late in the day to terminate the pregnancy. You may not want to even consider an abortion. At least one couple who have a child with Down's syndrome decided not to have an amniocentesis in two subsequent pregnancies. In the end it is your choice. But remember that you will "see" your baby on the sonogram just before the test, and are likely to be feeling the baby move about when the test results come in.

CHOOSING A DOCTOR FOR YOUR BABY

You will need to appoint a doctor to act as pediatrician from the moment your baby is born. Solicit names from your obstetrician and trusted friends. As you do your research, you may find that a particular doctor's name will keep popping up. While this doctor may be overworked and have less time for your baby, he or she may still offer the best care in your area. Check that name out first.

You can use some of the techniques you used earlier when evaluating your obstetric team. Write down general areas and issues that are important to you and use them as a basis for choosing the right doctor for your baby. With your list as a guide, you can interview each candidate and decide if the doctor's baby philosophy coincides with your own.

SAMPLE LIST OF BABY DOCTOR CRITERIA

- **Supports breast-feeding wholeheartedly (not all do)**
- **Has convenient calling hours**
- **Is conveniently located**
- **Has top-quality partners or back-up during vacation**
- **Will be on hand in the hospital to examine the baby after birth**
- **Is up-to-date on the latest pediatric trends**

NAMING YOUR BABY

This is perhaps the most important gift you will give to your baby, so choose carefully. There are several baby-name books on the bookshelves in stores (there is one in this series) or you may want to use a name from your family or a close friend. Narrow choices down by first looking at your surname. If it is one syllable, a longer first name will sound better (consider the difference between John Jones and Jonathan Jones). A short first name will be less cumbersome for a surname with more than one syllable (consider John Anderson and Jonathan Anderson). In general, try to avoid having the same number of syllables in both first and last names.

BABY EQUIPMENT

The Nursery and Layette

The decisions keep coming. Babies aren't particularly fussy about where they live or how they travel, nor do they care very much what they wear, as long as they are not wearing either too much or too little of it. *You* are the one who is eager to have everything just right. But no matter; the brouhaha of nursery and layette preparation helps to pass the time while you are waiting for the baby's arrival.

THE NURSERY

Zealous nursery preparations are often part of the last trimester when you feel a sudden surge of energy, commonly known as the "nesting instinct." You are coming in for the final stretch; your baby is sizable and active. His arrival is clearly visible on the horizon. Creating his environment will help you envision what life will be like when you are a family.

In the early weeks the baby will be asleep most of the time he is in his room. Later on, the nursery will also be a playroom with toy shelves and toys to play with. If you are going to have the room painted, consider choosing bright, primary colors. (If you want to do the work yourself, by the way, you should check with your doctor first about the likelihood of inhaling paint or other fumes which may not be advisable.) Babies love bright colors; indeed, research shows that newborns cannot even *see* soft pastels. But you may not want to look at a whole room painted red and blue, so you can accent pale walls with bright touches. In addition babies prefer patterns to solid colors, so you might consider using colorful wallpaper to decorate the walls.

Where will the baby sleep? Probably in a crib. A cradle is small and usable only in the first few months of life. Babies grow fast! If a friend or relative offers a cradle. you may wish to accept, if it is stable and sturdy, but don't purchase one because they are expensive and can be used for such a short time.

CRIBS AND CRIB MATTRESSES

Buying the crib and crib mattress are landmark decisions which can daunt expectant parents. In examining the cribs in a showroom you might want to look for cribs that:

- are sturdy and stable
- have adjustable mattress levels
- are on casters
- have short cornerposts (knobs are hazardous)
- have a convenient dropside mechanism (easy for you, but difficult for baby to maneuver)
- have plastic-covered teething guards on top rails

Crib mattresses are either made of urethane foam or have inner springs that are either pocketed or wire-tied; they must fit snugly into the crib. The urethane mattresses come in varying thicknesses, are lighter than the coil mattresses and usually are allergy-free.

If you are considering rehabilitating a secondhand shop "find" or borrowing a family heirloom, take extra care to make sure it is safe. Old cribs are notoriously unsafe. There should be a minimum amount of space between the slats so that your baby's head cannot get caught (the Consumer Product Safety Commission allows no more than $2\frac{3}{8}$ inches between slats). Make sure the crib is sturdy and stable with no missing screws or pieces, and when replacing the mattress make sure the new one fits snugly to avoid any danger of accidental suffocation. If the wood needs refinishing, use only nontoxic paints and finishes.

When you have bought the crib and set it up, take extra

BABY ESSENTIALS

100 newborn-size disposable diapers (or cloth equivalent)

4–6 stretch suits (fewer if weather is warm)

2–4 undershirts (more if weather is warm or very cold)

3 nightgowns or sleeping bags (lighter fabric in warm weather, heavier in cold weather)

1–3 sweaters

2 hats (knit for winter, or broad-brimmed for summer)

1–2 snowsuits

3 sets crib sheets

3 crib blankets

6 receiving blankets

1 contoured sponge for baby to lie on during bath

---

thought over where you place it in the room. For example, put it away from windows the baby might climb up to, and venetian blind cords that he might reach and wrap around his neck. Avoid putting toys in the crib that he can use as a boost in climbing out. A newborn cannot do these things, of course, but babies grow and acquire skills with astonishing speed. Before you know it, he will be climbing, and that is what causes accidents.

LAYETTE

This fancy word refers to the baby clothes, sheets and blankets the baby needs to get started in life. You will probably get lots of these as presents when the baby is born, and a relative may offer to give you the entire layette, which may either be simple or very elaborate. You really do not need much to start out with.

TIPS ON CAR SAFETY SEATS

BEFORE YOU BUY:

- Consider a convertible safety seat suitable for infant and toddler.
- Make sure it has a label stating that it meets or exceeds Federal Motor Vehicle Safety Standard 213.
- Make sure an adult can get the baby in and out with ease. Car seats that aren't used can't save lives.

AFTER PURCHASE:

- Follow the installation instructions carefully. Hook up the tether, if required.
- Make sure the harness is snug around the baby and that the car seat belt fits tightly around the restraint system.
- For small newborns, roll diapers or blankets for support.

CAR SEAT

This item should be at the top of your list in the last months of pregnancy. You can get by with almost nothing in the way of baby things, but if you drive a car, *you must have a car seat to take the baby home from the hospital and everywhere else you go after that.* Too often infants and children are killed and seriously injured in car accidents. Child restraint systems, when used properly, can greatly reduce this dreadful possibility.

THE PARENT CONSUMER

The car seat and crib are the only truly, absolutely essential accouterments a baby needs before birth. But in the course of the next few months and years, you will probably sink an unbelievable amount of money into such items as an infant seat, infant swing, stroller, playpen, walker, and more. Some are necessary, others are optional, all have safety features to be on the lookout for. Before making a purchase, check the consumer guides, ask your friends, compare prices, just as you would for any major purchase. But remember when it comes to the baby's things, the safety of the equipment must have priority over all.

Now, on with the show!

CHAPTER 4

Countdown and Lift-Off

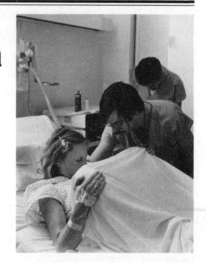

Τhe time has come to make final preparations for your baby's arrival; the excitement is palpable as you and your mate approach the last weeks. Childbirth class has begun and you are practicing breathing and relaxation techniques. In class you are also meeting other couples with whom you can commiserate and compare notes, falling into the normal social life of new parents. It is natural to seek the company of others who can share your experiences, concerns and triumphs.

Later, after the baby is born, your topics of conversation will center on your baby and her eating and sleeping patterns. But for now, you want to talk about how you feel and your preparations for the baby. If a classmate becomes a confidant, your conversation may turn to speculations and worries about the childbirth experience just ahead.

Continuing on this trail of important topics so crucial to you now, this chapter begins with the final preparations before the baby comes. Then, without further ado, we shall start labor, define what it is and describe how it progresses, and end, of course, with the triumph of childbirth.

Childbirth Checklist

MUSCLE PREP.

Do your Kegels. Your what? The Kegel is a conditioning exercise named after Arnold Kegel, a gynecologist who in

---

OTHER CONDITIONING EXERCISES

PELVIC ROCK

1. On hands and knees, arch your back like a cat, pointing pelvis upward, and tighten abdomen and buttocks. Return to level gradually.

2. Lying on your back on the floor, knees bent with feet on floor, flatten the lower back, pressing spine to the floor.

SQUATTING

Standing with feet comfortably apart with a straight spine, slowly lower yourself to squat, keeping heels on floor. To stand up, push up with your legs until knees are straight.

TAILOR PRESS

Sit with a straight back, soles of your feet together as close to your body as feels comfortable. Concentrate on gradually stretching thigh muscles so that your knees move closer to the floor.

---

the 1950s suggested that muscles around the vagina and rectum should be strengthened to combat urinary incontinence. The Kegel or perineal squeeze tones up the muscles that support the baby against gravity's pull and, when childbirth begins, must be relaxed. In addition, Kegels increase muscle control and circulation. If practice continues after the baby is born, they also promote healing and ease soreness. (Another dividend: enhanced sexual pleasure for both you and your mate.)

You can practice squeezing these muscles any time, anywhere: on the bus, putting on your makeup or reading the newspaper. But to ensure you don't forget, incorporate Kegels into your daily routine. Do a few sets each day, trying to hold each one for about ten seconds. It will get easier as the muscles strengthen.

SIB PREP.

You should tell an older child the big news about halfway through your pregnancy, when you begin to show and when everyone else knows about the new baby. Involve your child in baby preparations. Taking him along on prenatal doctor visits to hear the fetal heartbeat, reading aloud children's books about birth, and asking for "help" in getting baby things ready can help a child begin to accept a new sister or brother. Gauge what you do to your child's age and interest.

As your time nears, arrange for a relative or adult whom the child knows and likes to care for him while you are in the hospital. It is best if the child remains in his own environment. He will be less afraid that you are replacing him with this new baby. Tell him a "real-life story." Explain to him that you will be away for a few days, and that you *will* return, with a sister or brother. If the hospital allows siblings

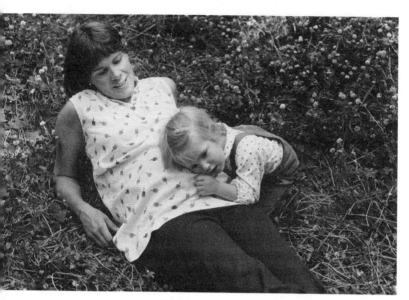
Big sister gets a first hearing of the baby that will change her life.

to visit, make sure he comes as often as possible and pack small presents for him to open when he arrives. If hospital policy forbids sibling visits, send those small presents home with notes about how much you love and miss him. (See Chapter 5 for some homecoming hints.)

HOSPITAL PREP.

Taking a tour of the maternity floor and the nursery will help prepare you for the experience to come. You can meet some of the staff, see the rooms and, if you have not already done so, ask questions about hospital policy.

Arranging preadmission to the hospital now will eliminate the hassle of filling out forms when labor has begun. Read the fine print in any medical consent form carefully before you sign.

PACKING FOR THE HOSPITAL

Labor Bag:

Your own pillow(s)
Lip balm
Talcum powder, tennis balls
  for massage
Favorite photo
Music
Camera, loaded with film
Lollipops
Newspapers, a favorite
  book to read aloud to
  pass the time

Hospital Case:

Nightgown, robe (with easy
  opening if you will be
  nursing)
Slippers
Toilet articles and hair dryer
Nursing bras (buy one size
  larger than your seven-
  months-pregnant size)
Something to read (not funny;
  laughing will be painful for
  a while)
List of friends' phone
  numbers
Baby blanket(s) and stretch
  suit; hat, snowsuit if
  weather is cold
Presents for older child

HOME PREP.

Cook meals ahead and store them in Ziploc freezer bags. The first two weeks at home, when you and the baby are adjusting, are confusing and exhausting. Shopping and planning for meals will be the last thing you feel like doing. Pulling a favorite dish out that you just have to thaw and heat is a morale boost that you deserve. To stretch out your frozen meal selection, collect take-out menus of restaurants that deliver and keep their phone numbers handy.

If your husband cannot take off much time from work after the baby comes, line up a relative or friend to help around the house. Most people do not need a baby nurse in the beginning; what they need is help in every other aspect of home life. Ask someone who is willing to keep the house while you tend the baby. Your helper should be someone who supports you as you learn how to be a mother, and also makes tactful suggestions at appropriate times.

LABOR: THE THREE STAGES

First Stage: Effacement and Dilation of the Cervix

The flattening or effacement and opening up of the cervix to ten centimeters, sometimes described as "five fingers," is the longest part of the whole process of childbirth. Sometimes the Braxton-Hicks contractions that precede labor have done some of the work of flattening out the cervix and opening it up. But labor that begins without a head start may go just as quickly. With a first pregnancy there is no way to predict how it will go. In subsequent pregnancies the history of a previous labor and delivery may be a rough guide, but surprises often happen.

HOW IT STARTS

Labor is usually mild at first, starting off with premenstrual-like symptoms while the uterus tenses up at regular intervals. False labor has a similar feeling, but the contractions occur at irregular intervals and go away if you walk around. These false alarms before true labor begins are disappointing and frustrating, especially if your due date has come and gone.

- Baby "lightens" or drops into your pelvis (up to two to three weeks before labor)
- Rupture of amniotic sac membranes or "waters breaking" (may also happen when labor is well established)
- Passing the tiny blood-stained mucous plug (may happen days before, at onset or during labor)

WHAT TO DO

If your waters break or contractions lasting about 45 seconds come every ten to 15 minutes, you must call your doctor. If you are experiencing pain or other worrisome symptoms, you should also feel free to check in with your doctor or midwife. A vaginal exam may be necessary to determine if your symptoms are truly labor.

If it is clear that you are in labor, your doctor will advise when you should come to the hospital. You should alert

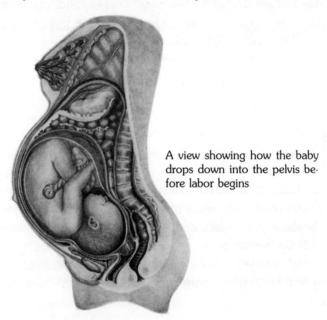

A view showing how the baby drops down into the pelvis before labor begins

your husband and tell him where to meet you. Once he is with you, he can help you time the length of your contractions and the time interval between them. (The time between contractions is measured from the beginning of one to the beginning of the next.) In a first pregnancy usually there is no need to rush to the hospital in the early stage of labor when contractions are mild and spaced far apart.

Slow, even breathing, inhaling through your nose and exhaling through your mouth will help you during early contractions. While you are waiting for your labor to get into full swing, you can pass the time by moving about. Taking a shower, washing your hair, smoothing on body lotion will help you relax. These efforts will also help you face the hard day's night ahead looking and feeling your best.

You are usually advised not to eat after labor has begun, but some doctors allow a little clear liquid like broth or sugar tea and crackers in the early part of the first stage. But keep in mind that it is particularly important to keep your bladder empty during labor, as a full one may increase discomfort and retard progress.

INDUCED LABOR

If you've not begun labor two weeks after your EDD, or doctors have reason to believe the placenta is not doing its job, your labor will probably be induced. The most common procedure is to break your amniotic waters and administer the drug oxytocin in an intravenous needle. Another catalyst for inducing labor is a synthetic hormone called prostaglandin which may be used as a suppository, gel, or a tablet. If your labor is induced, you may skip the early, easygoing phase of labor and contractions will be intense right from the start.

GETTING SET UP IN THE HOSPITAL

When you arrive, a nurse or physician will ask you questions about the onset of your labor and do a routine check of blood pressure and pulse, as well as an internal exam to see your progress thus far. Depending on your understanding with your medical team, you may then have an IV needle inserted into your hand to feed you fluid and medication.

And finally the nurse will attach the electronic fetal monitor to record the frequency and length of the contractions and track your baby's heartbeat. There are two types of fetal monitors: an external monitor which encircles your abdomen with straps or belts, and an internal monitor, which can be used after the membranes have ruptured, which attaches a tiny electrode to the baby's head.

Active Phase: From Four to Eight Centimeters

When you enter this level of labor, the fun of anticipation is over; this is serious business. An invisible wall goes up around you as you concentrate on riding out the storm of your labor. By now you are set up in the birthing room, birthing bed or old-fashioned labor room. Your contractions are more intense now, last longer and are three to five minutes apart. They require concentration and, when the initial slow breathing no longer helps, a different breathing pattern that is shallow and slightly accelerated will be needed. Internal exams to check your progress will be more frequent (be sure to request that the medical team wait until after a contraction has passed, because such an exam can intensify the pain).

WHAT IS A CONTRACTION AND WHY DOES IT HURT?

The muscles of the upper part of the uterus tense up, flattening and pulling back the cervix fibers. Contractions usually last anywhere from 45 to 90 seconds, rising to a peak halfway through and subside gradually during the remaining seconds. They are spaced farther apart in the beginning, around ten minutes. As labor progresses, the intervals shorten to five and then to two minutes apart. The intensity of the pressure in a contraction usually means that labor is progressing, because weak ones are not particularly effective. Women report different intensities of pain: some barely feel it, others experience strong pain.

No one knows the exact source of pain in contractions. Two possible causes are lack of oxygen in the uterine muscles and tense abdominal muscles interfering with uterine contractions. These theories about pain in childbirth directly correlate to the breathing and relaxation techniques taught in childbirth classes. Indeed, this training for childbirth has enabled thousands of women to control pain and reduce, if not eliminate entirely, pain medication required in labor.

A LABOR COACH'S GUIDE TO THE FIRST STAGE

- Speak encouraging words as often as possible
- Massage or apply counterpressure to her aching back
- Help her to relax
- Breathe with her
- Speak up if her preferences about procedures are overlooked by hospital staff
- Wipe her brow, feed her ice chips
- Ignore her hostility in transition, remind her the end is near
- Help her know how much time is left in a contraction

TYPES OF MEDICATIONS AND USES

Type:	Use:
Synthetic hormonal (Pitocin)	To induce or strengthen labor, stop bleeding after delivery
Tranquilizers	To lower tension and anxiety in labor
Analgesics (Demerol)	To ease backache and take edge off pain
Regional anesthesia (block)	To numb centers of pain for procedures like forceps delivery or cesarean birth
General anesthesia	For emergency cesarean procedure

Transition: A Short Tour Through Hell

The end of the first stage of labor, when the cervix opens the last two or three centimeters, is a dramatic phase called transition. Contractions are now at their highest intensity and come every 90 seconds or so. The interval between the end of one contraction and the start of another is only about 30 seconds. The turbulent nature of transition ensures that it is relatively short in duration. Hostile words and a short temper usually announce that you have reached the beginning of the end. You may also tremble, or feel nauseous and sleepy during the short breaks between contractions.

As you progress toward full dilation, you will feel increased pressure on your rectum and feel an urge to push. It is better not to push until the cervix is fully dilated. Until the midwife or attending doctor tells you it is time to push, you must control your muscles (remember all those Kegels?). A switch in your breathing will help, too: Punctuate your shallow panting with an occasional forceful blowing out of air.

Delivery: The Second Stage

Once you get the go-ahead to push, you can bear down with each contraction, working with your uterus to get the baby through the birth canal. Depending on the baby's size and your pelvic structure, this stage can take a few contractions or a couple of hours. The baby's head should rotate and relieve the pressure on your back, and then move down between your pubic bone and your tailbone. As the head

A husband-coach pitches in during labor.

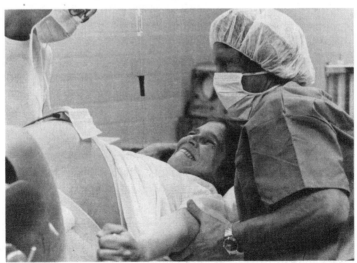

CESAREAN BIRTH

Although the labor we describe in this chapter is going swimmingly, we must interrupt to warn that childbirth does not always end as planned. According to the National Center for Health Statistics, in 1984 about 21 percent per 100 deliveries, or about one baby in five, were delivered by cesarean, up from just under 5 percent per 100 in 1965.

Most new parents are grateful and relieved when a cesarean has rescued their baby from danger. Sometimes the reasons for an operation are clear; but all too often, the attending doctors may decide without involving the new parents and explaining the change in delivery plans. Suddenly the birth they prepared for so eagerly is out of their control. Though they are delighted that their baby is healthy, parents are likely to be disappointed or feel as if they had failed.

You don't always have to accept a cesarean as inevitable, though. If your doctor says at a prenatal visit that your pelvis is too small, you can have another doctor examine you and get a second opinion. If your labor is moving too slowly, you can try walking around to stimulate contractions or increasing your fluid intake either with an IV or orally. If you have had a cesarean birth, and are pregnant again, you may be able to labor this time (see VBAC section in Chapter 3).

COMMON REASONS FOR CESAREANS

1. Feto-cephalopelvic disproportion (50-pound words that mean the mother's pelvis is too small for the baby, or the baby is too large)
2. Lack of progress in labor, weak or infrequent contractions
3. Baby is breech (feet first)
4. Fetal distress: irregular heartbeat shown on monitor
5. Previous cesarean birth

A cesarean birth is abdominal surgery that is performed in a regular operating room. If you have epidural anesthesia (an anesthetic injected into the base of the spine), you will be able to be alert and awake during your baby's birth. Seeing your baby born will go a long way relieving your frustration that you could not deliver vaginally. In emergency situations there will not be time to put in a regional block, and general anesthesia will be given.

Two incisions are made, one in the abdomen, one in the uterus. When the baby and later the placenta are lifted out, you may feel some pressure and nausea. After the baby is duly examined, you will probably be able to spend a few minutes with her. Then your husband will go with the pediatrician down to the nursery while the doctor sews the incisions, which will take about half an hour. You will spend time in the recovery room and it will be a while before you see either baby or husband.

clears these obstacles, it will become visible at the height of a contraction and eventually crown. In a few more contractions you will usually be able to push out the head, shoulders and body. The obstetrician will probably perform an episiotomy, an incision to widen the opening of the vagina, and you may have to hold back on pushing during a contraction for this to be done or to avoid tearing the stretched skin of the vagina. This can be hard because the urge to push is almost irresistible.

Many women are relieved of pain when the pushing starts. Instead of coping with pain by using the passive role of relaxation, a woman often finds the pressure she exerts to force the baby out anesthetizing. Unfortunately other women, because the baby does not rotate properly, experience yet more back labor pain.

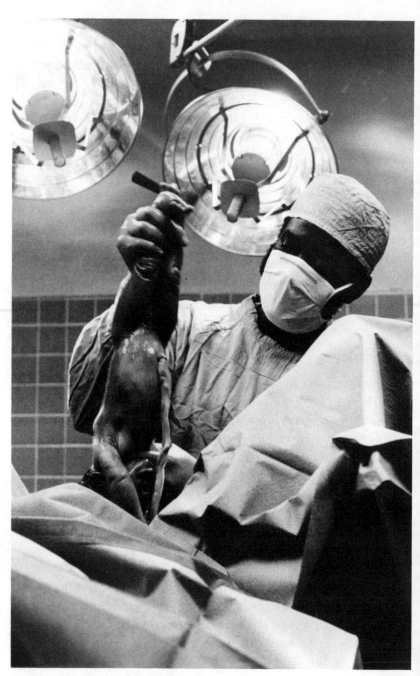

It's a real, live, healthy baby girl!

In this stage of labor a woman must muster all the strength she has left, particularly if the first stage has taken a very long time. Pushing is very hard work and requires its very own breathing pattern and body position. The tilted angle in a birthing bed or chair enlists the aid of gravity and can make the job easier. However the hospital delivery table forces you to lie on your back, so you must pull yourself up to push.

BREATHING PATTERN FOR PUSHING

As a contraction begins, inhale deeply through the nose and exhale; then take in another breath and hold it for 20 to 30 seconds while you bear down. You will need to exhale and quickly take another breath, then hold it while you push. A third breath may be necessary if the contraction lingers. Breathe normally between contractions.

A LABOR COACH'S GUIDE TO THE SECOND PHASE

- Give progress reports, praise and encouragement often
- Remind her to breathe deeply
- Support her shoulders during each contraction or adjust pillows so that she is propped up for pushing
- Be ready to pant with her through a contraction, if she must pause in her pushing for an episiotomy to be made
- Keep loaded camera ready to capture baby's birth

The Third Stage of Labor

The placenta, so important to the baby only seconds ago, now is useless. A few mild contractions will help detach it from the uterus and slip it through the vaginal opening. The third stage of labor is easier, but after delivering the baby you are, quite understandably, shaky. Adrenaline will help you through the last, essential part of your baby's birth. Immediately your hormones shift gears and additional mild contractions will continue, in order to close the open blood vessels where the placenta was lodged.

You Did It!

The labor and delivery of your baby is finished, at least on paper. When you actually go through childbirth, you should be proud of your achievement. You must not tie yourself down to any one scenario. Labor and delivery have all sorts of unexpected twists and turns that you cannot anticipate or control. That is why it is so important to have

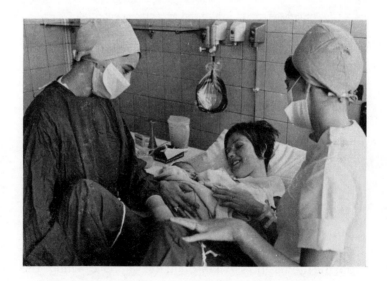

WHAT HAPPENS IMMEDIATELY AFTER BIRTH

Mother:	Baby:
Nurse massages uterus externally	Cord clamped and cut
Local anesthetic is administered and episiotomy sewn up (with stitches that will gradually dissolve)	Nose and throat suctioned
	Weighed, cleaned and footprinted
Sucks on lollipop or ice chips and rests	Eye drops, Vitamin K shot given
May breast-feed and hold baby	Physical Apgar test

skilled sympathetic professionals supporting you through each stage of the process.

A commitment to a drug-free labor can be eroded by hours of difficult labor, or the baby may get into trouble and suddenly your carefully planned, drug-free childbirth becomes an emergency cesarean requiring general anesthesia. Never grade yourself on how close you stick to a specific plan. Whatever else may have happened in labor, you were able to reach the finish line; you and your baby have made it through together.

CHAPTER 5

Firsthand Experience

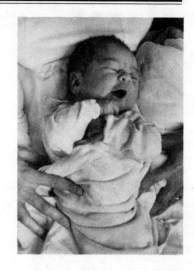

Now we can adjust our paper telescope to focus on the moment you have been waiting and preparing for these last nine months: holding and looking at your baby. If you plan to nurse, you will put him to your breast for the first time. Before birth your relationship with your baby is a strange mix of intimate separateness. Sight unseen (sonograms don't really count!), the two of you are connected by a cord that means life or death to him and the promise of the future to you. Communication is confined to him pummeling your internal organs while he listens to your thumping heartbeat and the gurglings of your stomach.

When the baby is born, you can feast your eyes on him and examine every line and curve of his precious body. The baby, in turn, has a chance to drink in the strange new world that suddenly surrounds him. In these early minutes and hours he has already begun the awesome task of babyhood: discovering the giant human world outside the womb. Isn't it wonderful that the gentleness of your hands can be his first lesson in life.

IN THE HOSPITAL

After Delivery

The amount of time you spend with your new baby immediately after delivery will depend on how you feel, on the baby's health and on hospital policy. Hospitals that encourage family-centered birth experiences are likely to give parents an uninterrupted hour soon after birth. Unless you have made other arrangements with your medical team, the baby will be "processed" by experienced hands with astounding speed, and the three of you will be left alone. During the first hour after birth babies are usually quiet, but alert in a so-called sensitive period when some experts believe babies have heightened awareness. After that, babies fall asleep.

PHOTO TIP: *Before the hospital staff leave you alone, have a nurse take your first family portrait; take shots of your birth attendants as well. This is a very special moment, one you will want to remember. Years later you will be able to show and tell your child the story of his birth.*

In the excitement and exhaustion of birth, you are not exactly your old self. You are euphoric, drained and dazed, but not at all sleepy—all at the same time! If you are feeling particularly shaky, you may not be able to hold the baby very successfully. Let him lie on your chest or nestle in the crook of your arm, supported with pillows. Give your husband a chance to hold him, too. You and he should begin now sharing the baby, a conscious policy of mutual responsibility and trust that cannot begin too early in the baby's life.

If, after only a few minutes, the baby is whisked away to the nursery and you are rolled down to your hospital bed, or if medical circumstances delay your time with the baby, do not fret that he will suffer irreparable damage.

Postpartum portrait of the medical team with mother and baby

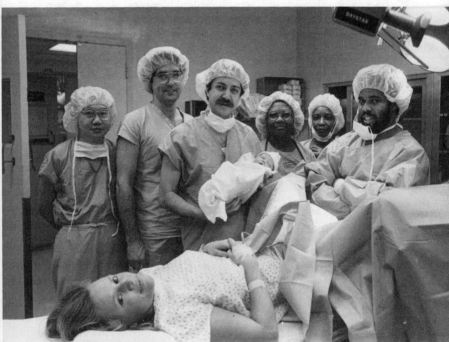

Though the first hour after birth is prime time to spend with your baby, the days, weeks and years that lie ahead will provide ample opportunities to build a close relationship with him.

Indeed, it will likely take some time before you feel really close to your baby. Bonding is a slow, step-by-step process that lasts a lifetime. It may get off to a slower start than you first imagined. After childbirth you are often depleted and unable to muster the strength to experience strong emotions. Feelings will wait on the sidelines until you have recovered with a nap or a night's rest.

As you begin to regain your strength, you rejoice that your great ordeal is done, and that the baby's body is as it should be, with no details overlooked. (Don't worry if his head has an odd shape or if he looks a bit wrinkled; all that will change soon.) You are electrified, and perhaps overwhelmed, at the prospect of mothering this little baby. Suddenly what was a hazy picture in pregnancy comes into sharp focus. Two tasks lie clearly ahead: Finding out who your baby is and learning how to respond to him.

Rooming-In

Having your baby with you is the only way to bond with him; you must spend time discovering who he is and how to give him what he needs. Whether you start in the hospital or wait until you get home is not particularly crucial, but the ground has to be covered at some point. And sooner is probably better than later. Rooming-in at the hospital offers you a safe, secure way to learn about your baby's behavior and how to take care of him. Other experienced mothers and nursery nurses are excellent teachers who can guide you through the mysteries of disposable diapering and nursing. If you plan to breast-feed, rooming-in is almost an essential in order to get baby and you used to it.

Hospitals vary in their policy on how much time they allow babies to live in with the mother. Some allow 24-hour togetherness; others daytime rooming-in, with an optional 2:00 A.M. feeding. Daytime hours can be limited: Babies often must be in the nursery during visiting hours and pediatric rounds.

Don't be dissuaded from having the baby in with you by well-meaning nurses or relatives who think he will tire you by crying when you want to be sleeping. Most babies sleep a great deal in the first week, when they are not disturbed by other babies crying. Best of all, if the baby is in with you, you can check on him constantly whenever you need reassurance that he is really there and perfectly all right. The early days of motherhood are filled with tiny anxieties of this kind and with the baby close to you, you can dispel them and relax.

Recovery After Vaginal Birth

As we have said, you will have a ballooning middle for awhile. It should deflate considerably after the first week or two. The pregnancy machine which has been built up over a nine-month period must be taken apart. The postpartum period is full of radical changes: Your uterus shrinks, your blood volume is cut by a third, excess fluid drops off and your hormones shift gears. The wounds from the birth, both inside the uterus where the placenta was attached, and the external episiotomy incision must heal; stretched out muscles and tissues must gradually regain their tone.

Recovering from a Cesarean Birth

One very good reason for choosing not to have your baby with you constantly is if you feel rotten. A cesarean birth is abdominal surgery and you will recover more slowly from it than other women do after vaginal childbirth. If you are given general anesthesia, it will take you some two weeks to feel the way your vaginal delivery sisters felt after about an hour.

Every move you make that requires the help of a stomach muscle—clearing your throat, shifting position, getting out of bed, or walking, for example—is very painful. A cough is truly excruciating.

Depression is common, a reaction to the continuing pain and to the disappointment of a birth plan gone awry. A sense of failure is hard to escape, particularly when the cesarean mother looks at other mothers in the maternity ward who sail through their recovery after vaginal birth.

Mothering is a terrible struggle in those first few days.

COPING WITH CESAREAN RECOVERY

- As soon as you can, move around and walk even though it is painful. You have got to get your blood and intestines moving again.
- Consider pain medication to help you through the first couple of days. It is easier to move if it doesn't hurt so much.
- If you have to cough, hold a pillow tightly over your abdomen for support.
- Also practice tightening those muscles, using the same pillow for support.
- Consider breast-feeding: It is a morale boost. It will help you bond with the baby and heal your uterus, too. (Though it may hurt as the uterine muscles contract, what's a little more pain?)
- Rest and sleep as much as possible. The baby can wait.
- Use the "pregnant method" for getting out of bed: Roll onto your side and push yourself up with your arm to a sitting position.
- Do small, gentle exercises to increase circulation: Move around whatever doesn't hurt.
- Express your feelings. The emotions you feel are real; bottling them up inside will delay your recovery.
- Talk to your husband about how you feel and find out how he is coping. Sharing a burden makes it easier to shoulder.

You aren't able to maneuver holding your baby very well, and may have to ask a nurse to help you switch from one breast to another. God forbid you should have to move to reach for a bottle or a diaper. Rooming-in must wait until you feel better. But you *will* feel better. Time (and tips) heal all wounds.

Hospital Miscellany

NEWBORN CARE

If the birth has been a hard one, your baby may be placed in an incubator for a few hours to recuperate; if he is premature, the incubator will be essential to provide the warmth he needs for optimal growth. As his digestive tract is immature, he will also need to be fed via intravenous

A neonatal nurse cuddles premature twins.

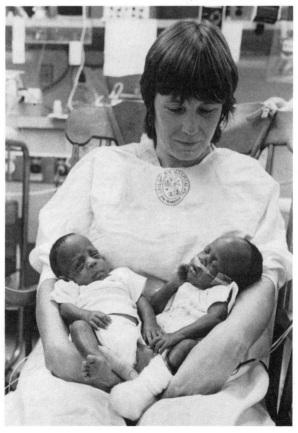

needle or tube. These machines and wires help preemies through the transitional growth period that would otherwise have been the third trimester of pregnancy.

Hospitals usually offer class instruction on handling new babies. It is strongly advised that all new mothers, as soon as they are able, go to classes while they are still in the hospital. A nursery nurse will demonstrate with one of the babies in the nursery how to diaper, bathe and swaddle a newborn. Other important topics include taking a temperature and bottle feeding. Bring a pillow to sit on and watch an experienced hand in action.

SWOLLEN SEXUAL ORGANS

Don't be alarmed if your new baby, exquisitely tiny in every other detail, has somewhat larger sexual organs than you would expect. This is a natural effect of the hormones that have been circulating in your bloodstream which he had shared with you. It will pass off very quickly.

JAUNDICE

Babies in the nursery sometimes have a yellowish skin color that looks like a tan from a Florida vacation. The yellow tint comes from a bile pigment called bilirubin which is supposed to be broken down by the liver and then flushed out through the intestines. Babies' livers are immature and may be slow to process the bilirubin which in turn colors the skin.

Jaundice usually appears the third day and disappears after a week or ten days. A heel prick blood test will determine the level of excess bilirubin. Hospital policies vary, but if your baby's blood shows more than 15 milligrams per 100 milliliters of serum in the blood, he will probably be put under "bili lights" for 12 to 72 hours. These lights help to decompose the bilirubin and bring the baby's bili count down to a safer level. Periodic blood checks will determine how long he has to stay under the lights.

AT HOME

If You Have an Older Child

You may want to make bringing the baby home from the hospital a major family event. If your older child can participate, she will feel included and less likely to suspect you are replacing her with a newer model. Or you may want to bring the baby home while the sibling is out of the house, so that you and the baby can be calmly situated when they first meet. Any nervousness and confusion getting the baby settled in his new home may detract from that important first hands-on meeting.

It is important that your older child, however young, have a chance to hold and fondle the baby. Even if you strongly suspect that the first caress will be much more like a hit or a poke, do not communicate this fear to her. But be ready to intervene at the last second. Once they have met, plan to ignore the baby for a while and devote your attention to your older child.

CAUTION: *As you settle in, you will not be able to leave these two new sibs alone even for a second. Either resentment or clumsiness may turn a hug into a painful experience. Without warning your older child may decide to feed the baby Legos for lunch. If toddler is around, have the baby with you wherever you go. Life will be easier as you learn to sprout eyes in the back of your head!*

Overwhelmed and Overtired

Help when you first come home is invaluable, but temporary. After a few days or a week, your husband will usually have to go back to work or your relative must leave you (but depending on who it is and the help you get, you may be relieved to be alone).

New mothers often feel nervous when they bring their babies home from the hospital, in awe of their new-found responsibilities. Decisions that seem crucial must be made every day of the baby's life. Sometimes it may seem like too much to handle. Lack of sleep stretches patience to the breaking point. Every night you must wake up once, if not twice, to feed your charge. It is all too easy to run yourself into the ground, sapping the energy and stamina so necessary for mothering.

COMBAT FATIGUE

- **Nap when your baby naps (phone off the hook)**
- **Get weekly help (someone to clean your house, run errands, etc.)**
- **Get away from the baby by hiring sitters for short periods several times a week**

As you go through each day, try to remember that your baby is sturdier than he looks. No mother always does the right thing. The baby will thrive if you use a commonsense approach to his care. If he is wetting half a dozen diapers, and soiling at least one a day, he is on the right track. He will cry to alert you that something is not right—though you may not be able to fix it!

GETTING SETTLED

The first few days at home are often difficult. The baby's schedule of eating and sleeping is usually erratic, and you probably don't feel comfortable with all the crying he does. To head off his crying, you try to anticipate what he will need next and keep a careful eye on the clock. But it is difficult to discern a pattern of eating and sleeping and what works one time will not necessarily work the next. Be prepared to be frustrated for awhile. His needs will not settle down for two to three weeks, at least.

You will also discover that he cries not only when he is hungry or tired, but for other reasons that are more difficult to explain. If you are nervous, angry or upset, the baby may catch your mood. Other culprits may be overstimulation or pain from gas or colic. Often you won't know why he is crying (and if the baby could speak, he would probably not be able to tell you), but you keep on trying different answers until he stops, either because you find the solution or because he finally drops off to sleep.

THE EARLY EVENING BLUES

Babies often choose 5:00 P.M. or so to be fussy, though some start earlier or later. Whenever his personal buzzer sounds and the baby starts driving you crazy, you will often find that you are a) tired from the day's efforts and b) trying to straighten the house or make dinner.

TIP: *Stop what you are doing, pull out your restaurant delivery menus, and sit down with the baby. Many mothers find, when all else fails, that drinking a beer or a small glass of wine at this hour helps them get through this difficult time (and helps their milk let down, too, if they are nursing).*

Developing a Mental Checklist

The art of mothering hinges on knowing what time it is. If you do not already own a watch, it should be the first item on your shopping list (one that can be read in the dark is especially useful now). You need to check the time whenever the baby does anything: You want to know when he nurses, begins to fuss, starts or finishes a nap, when he goes to bed and when he wakes up.

Developing a list to run through will help you to crack

SAMPLE SITUATION

Your baby has been awake and content for a while and now begins to fuss.

1. Check the time since he last slept. If you suspect he is about ready for a nap or bedtime, you should run down the rest of the checklist, to make sure he is ready for sleep. If you doubt that he is sleepy, run down the list looking for the solution to his crying in the order that seems appropriate at the time.

2. Decide how long since he has been fed. If he is hungry, feed him. If it has been a couple of hours since he has eaten, see if he has interest in a bottle or your breast. You don't want to put the baby to bed on a near empty stomach as he might wake up hungry after only a short nap.

3. Check his diaper.

4. Change his position from back to tummy or vice versa. Change the scenery. Maybe he is just bored.

5. Have the cocktail-hour blues struck? Maybe he needs you to sit down and hold him. Or strap him to your chest in a cloth carrier as you move about.

---

the code and solve the mysteries of who your baby is and what he needs. Sometimes you will run through your repertoire and find that you are no closer to making your baby stop crying. You will probably become frustrated and possibly frightened because your best effort is not enough. It may be that he is feeling irritable and just needs to be left alone to cry it out.

Emotional Fallout of Mothering

DEPRESSION

Standing side by side, next to your elation at having a newborn baby, are other rather negative feelings which are just as normal as the positive ones. Depression may come the first week after birth when the postpartum blues hit. Triggered by overall physical weakness and hormonal shifts now that you are not pregnant anymore, the depression may intensify if your self-esteem is low or you feel unattractive. You may resent that your baby is now getting the attention that was centered on you when you were pregnant.

Now is when you bring out those clothes you bought in Chapter 2 and continue Chapter 3's practice of rewarding yourself for each day's job well done. Motherhood in general is more difficult than pregnancy and mothering a newborn is the most difficult of all.

CLAUSTROPHOBIA AND ISOLATION

You are indoors too much, confined to quarters with the baby. As soon as your pediatrician says he can go outside, try getting out, even for a walk around the block. Happily, the baby is small and portable (though often the accessories you carry for an afternoon out may seem as if you are going away for the weekend!), and does not care where he is as long as he is with you.

Unless it is very cold out, you should be able to take him anywhere you have the energy to go. Check with your pediatrician if you are in doubt as to the advisability of venturing out. If it is cold outside, dress him warmly in a snowsuit and hat, but don't overdo it. Young babies cannot regulate their body temperature very well and get very red and hot if dressed too warmly.

If you cannot get out, get sitters in. Another remedy is to invite friends with similar interests over for a visit. Commiseration and company will help.

RESENTMENT AND FRUSTRATION

You may also feel resentment because you are slave to a baby who does not yet respond affectionately to you, despite his demands for endless attention. You feel frustrated when the jobs in and out of the house that were so easy and quick to do now are a big deal. No longer can you just run out to the grocery for eggs and milk—it has become a major production. Ditto for an evening out: not only must you find a sitter who knows what she is doing around a baby, you must also give her endless instructions. And then, of course, you find it hard not to worry about how the baby is doing once you are out for the evening.

RX FOR EMOTIONAL STRESS

The reward system that we have talked about all along should be used as a ladder you can climb to lift you out of the roiling negative currents of your mind and heart. What you choose should be realistic for your pocketbook (and nonfattening).

- **Regular evenings out with sitters booked month by month, say every Wednesday and Saturday, 8:00–10:00 P.M.**
- **Regular weekly afternoon get-together with a friend and her small baby (remember your childbirth class friends)**
- **Make a date to be with your husband, turn off the phone and focus on each other (see below)**
- **Make time each day for yourself to do what you like: reading, sewing, talking on the phone, etc.**

Sex After Childbirth

Doctors usually advise a standard six-week waiting period before resuming intercourse, the time it will probably take your stitches and soreness to heal. If you find sex unexpectedly painful, there may be an undissolved stitch or an unhealed area; consult your doctor for help at once. The method of contraception depends on your own preference, unless you are nursing. Nursing mothers should use barrier methods such as diaphragm with jelly or condoms and avoid the Pill, which reduces the milk supply and passes hormones to the baby. If a diaphragm is chosen, it must be fitted (or refitted) at the postpartum checkup.

You may not care about sex for a while after childbirth. Physiological and emotional changes can have a variety of temporary effects on your sex life, not necessarily positive. Hormone activity in nursing mothers make them particularly susceptible to a lowering of sexual interest and appetite. If you are feeling fragile, exhausted or alienated from your mate, you can rekindle the fire slowly by snuggling, hugging and kissing. These are fundamental ways of recharging emotional batteries and restoring harmony with each other.

If you are having trouble in your marriage right now, it may be that the lines of communication are down. Reread the last part of Chapter 2 on communication and sex; the books in the Adult Needs section of the Bibliography have wise counsel to offer, too.

You've Come a Long Way with This Baby!

Remember when the baby was no bigger than the dot of an "i"? The process of becoming a parent is painful and difficult; but (as somebody's mother probably said) nothing worth doing is easy. Gradually, the baby has grown into both your lives until it is hard to remember what life was like without him. Now you are a family, bound intimately together.

Before your eyes, the miracle you have begun will continue to unfold, bringing new challenges and joy. Nurturing your baby as he grows with each passing day, the seemingly endless job of mothering, is surely the most important work you will ever do.

Bibliography

GENERAL

The Maternity Sourcebook: 230 Basic Decisions for Pregnancy, Birth and Baby Care, by Matthew and Wendy Lesko (New York: Warner Books, 1984).

PREPARING FOR PARENTHOOD

Planning Ahead for Pregnancy: Dr. Cherry's Guide to Health, Fitness and Fertility, by Sheldon H. Cherry, M.D. (New York: Viking, 1987).

Letters to a Child Never Born, by Oriana Fallaci (New York: Doubleday, 1976).

A Baby?. . .Maybe, by Elizabeth M. Whelan, Sc.D. (New York: Bobbs-Merrill, 1976).

LIFE IN THE WOMB

A Child is Born, by Lennart Nilsson (New York: Dell, 1976).

The First Nine Months of Life, by Geraldine Lux Flanagan (New York: Simon & Schuster, 1962).

The Secret Life of the Unborn Child, by Thomas Verny (New York: Summit, 1981).

HAVING BABIES LATER IN LIFE

Having a Baby After 30, by Elisabeth Bing and Libby Colman (New York: Bantam, 1975).

Parents After Thirty, by Murray Kappelman and Paul Ackerman (New York: Wideview Books, 1981).

The Pregnancy After 30 Workbook, by Gail Brewer (Emmaus, PA: Rodale Press, 1978).

Pregnancy After 35, by Carole McCauley (New York: Pocket Books, 1976).

BEAUTY IN PREGNANCY

How to Look Good and Feel Great, by Bonnie Estridge (Secaucus, NJ: Chartwell Books, 1982).

Newborn Beauty, by Wende D. Bates (New York: Bantam, 1981).

The Pregnant Woman's Beauty Book, by Gloria Natale (New York: William Morrow, 1980).

NUTRITION IN PREGNANCY

Eating Right: Before, During and After Pregnancy, by Elizabeth Whelan (New York: American Baby Books, 1982).

Nourishing Your Unborn Child: Nutrition and Natural Foods in Pregnancy, by Phyllis Williams (New York: Avon, 1975).

EXERCISE IN PREGNANCY

The Jane Fonda Workout Book For Pregnancy, Birth and Recovery, by Femmy DeLyser (New York: Simon & Schuster, 1982).

Moving Through Pregnancy, by Elisabeth Bing (New York: Bantam, 1976).

Suzy Prudden's Pregnancy and Back-to-Shape Exercise Program, by Suzy Prudden (New York: Workman, 1982).

ADULT NEEDS IN PREGNANCY AND PARENTING

Making Love During Pregnancy, by Elisabeth Bing and Libby Colman (New York: Bantam, 1977).

The Private Life of Parents: How to Take Care of Yourself and Your Partner While Raising Happy, Healthy Children—A Complete Survival Guide, by Roberta Plutzik and Maria Laghi (New York: Everest House, 1983).

Sex, by Michael Carrera (New York: Crown Publishers, 1981).

BIRTH PLAN ALTERNATIVES

Birth Without Violence by Frederick Leboyer (New York: Knopf, 1980).

The Complete Book of Midwifery, by Barbara Brennan and Joan Rattner Heilman (New York: E.P. Dutton, 1979).

The Rights of the Pregnant Father: How to Have an Easier, Healthier Hospital Birth Together, by Valmai Howe Elkins (New York: Two Continents Publishing Group, 1976).

Shared Childbirth: A Guide to Family Birth Centers, by Philip Sumner and Celeste Phillips (St. Louis: C. V. Mosby, 1982).

CHILDBIRTH METHODS

Awake and Aware: Participating in Childbirth Through Psychoprophylaxis, by Irwin Chabon (New York: Delacorte, 1974).

Childbirth Without Fear, by Dr. Grantly Dick-Read (New York: Harper & Row, 1959).

The Complete Book of Pregnancy and Childbirth, by Sheila Kitzinger (New York: Knopf, 1980).

A Husband-Coached Childbirth, by Dr. Robert Bradley (New York: Harper & Row, 1974).

Methods of Childbirth, by Constance Bean (New York, Dolphin Books, 1982).

Six Practical Lessons for an Easier Childbirth, by Elisabeth Bing (New York: Bantam, 1969).

Thank You, Dr. Lamaze, by Marjorie Karmel (New York: Dolphin, 1965).

CESAREAN BIRTH

Cesarean Childbirth, by Christine Coleman Wilson and Wendy Roe (New York: Signet, 1980).

Cesarean Birth Experience, by Bonnie Donovan (Boston: Beacon, 1977).

Silent Knife, by Nancy Wainer Cohen and Lois Estner (South Hadley, MA: J.F. Bergen Publishers, 1983).

PREMATURE BIRTH

Born Early, by Dr. Mary Ellen Avery and Georgia Litwack (Boston: Little Brown, 1983).

Premature Babies: A Handbook for Parents, by Sherri Nance (New York: Arbor House, 1982).

ADJUSTING TO BABY

New Parenthood: The First Six Weeks, by Cecilia Worth with Anna Marie Brooks (New York: McGraw-Hill, 1985).

When the New Baby Comes, I'm Moving Out (a child's cartoon book), by Martha Alexander (New York: Dutton, 1979).

Index

PICTURE CREDITS

p. 10 Martin M. Rotker—Taurus Photos, Inc. 16 Hazel Hankin—Stock Boston
17 Maternity Center Association 21 Jean-Claude Lejeune—Stock Boston 22
Maternity Center Association 30 Jim Harrison—Stock Boston 35 Fredrik D.
Bodin—Stock Boston 38 Maternity Center Association 45 Nancy Durrell
McKenna—Photo Researchers, Inc. 54 Eric Kroll—Taurus Photos, Inc. 57 Peter
Vandermark—Stock Boston 60 Maternity Center Association 65 Suzanne
Szasz—Photo Researchers, Inc. 68 Chester Higgins, Jr.—Photo Researchers, Inc.
70 Laimute E. Druskis—Taurus Photos, Inc. 72 Mimi Forsyth—Monkmeyer
Press 74 Eric Kroll—Taurus Photos, Inc. 79 Karen Preuss—Taurus Photos, Inc.